1

Table of Contents

INTRODUCTION

Hello there! Thank you for joining us. Set off on a life-altering quest for self-

awareness. In this workbook, you will embark on a quest to rethink what it means to be successful and live life to the fullest. In today's fast-paced world, it's easy to feel overwhelmed by societal conventions, expectations, and obligations. Amidst the chaos, though, is a chance for you to make your life what you want it to be: true to who you are and everything you believe in. This workbook will show you the way to a life that is rich with purpose, happiness, and fulfilment. Each chapter is filled with insightful advice, motivational strategies, and actionable activities that will help you become an expert in your own life and build the life you've always dreamed of. No matter where you are in your journey towards self-discovery, more harmony in your life, or simply a stronger sense of connection to the universe, this workbook is here to help. That being said, jump in headfirst with an adventurous spirit. The power to transform your life and make a lasting impact lies within these pages, so dive in and discover yourself. Is an amazing voyage something you're interested in? Now we're going to do it. --- By inspiring readers to take action and realize their dreams, this opening part lays the

**groundwork for the remainder
of the workbook.**

- **CHAPTER 1: Defining
Your Ideal Lifestyle**

Establishing Your Perfect Way
of Life Envision a life where you
look forward to each morning

with anticipation, knowing that you will have a day full of experiences that satisfy you. For you, what constitutes the perfect way of life? We go off on an adventure of self-discovery in this chapter to find the plan for your dreams.

1.1 Contemplating Your Principles A person's priorities, behaviors, and decision-making are all shaped by their basic set of values. Think about the things that are important to you. What about bonding with loved ones, expressing one's creativity, going on adventures, or feeling free? The first step in creating a life that is true to who you are is gaining an awareness of your beliefs.

1.2 Creating the Ideal Day for You Imagine, in your mind's eye, the most ideal day ever. When did you wake up? Tell me what you're up to. Might I ask who you're accompanying? To better understand what contributes to your joy and fulfilment in life, try visualizing your perfect dreams

1.3 Deliberately Establishing Objectives Now that you know what kind of life you want, the next step is to make it a reality by establishing concrete objectives. How can you make your dream a reality? Achieving any objective, be it the launch of a new pastime, the exploration of faraway lands, or the strengthening of existing relationships, is a step closer to realizing your full potential.

1.4 Being Open to Change and Adaptable Embrace change and stay adaptive as you begin your journey of self-discovery. Your perfect way of living could change as you progress through life. Embracing new experiences and chances allows you to gracefully and resiliently manage life's twists and turns.

1.5 Developing an Attitude of Gratitude An abundant existence is built upon an attitude of gratitude. Every day, stop what you're doing and give thanks for all the good things in your life. You may improve your life in every way—attitude, joy, and abundance—by learning to be grateful.

1.6 Taking Action: Making a Manifesto for Your Perfect Lifestyle Make a public proclamation of your beliefs, aspirations, and ideal way of life by crafting an Ideal Lifestyle Manifesto before proceeding. If you want to find your life's true calling and follow your passions, then this manifesto is for you. ---

In this first chapter, we build the basis for readers to explore their values and goals in depth, which will help them create a life that is authentic to who they are.

- **CHAPTER 2: Setting Goals for a Fulfilling Life**

Achieving Your Life's Purposes
As we go through life, having clear and attainable goals serves as a compass to help us stay on track and achieve our aspirations. What follows is an examination of the significance of goal-setting as a tool for achieving a meaningful and satisfying life.

2.1 Why Setting Goals Is Crucial

Setting and working towards goals motivates us to excel in all areas of our lives and helps us achieve our full potential. They make our dreams a reality by providing us with direction, inspiration, and clarity. Discover your limitless potential and design a life that fulfils your wildest dreams by establishing ambitious yet attainable objectives.

2.2 Aiming with the SMART Framework Use the SMART framework—specific, measurable, achievable, relevant, and time-bound—to make sure your goals are practical and fruitful. You may achieve your goals more quickly and with more clarity if you follow this framework, which will also help you stay focused and accountable. 2.3 Determining Your Primary Concentrations Before you set any goals, take stock of your life and make a list of everything that matters most to you. Each facet of your life—your health and fitness, your profession and finances, your relationships, your personal development, and your leisure—is critical to your overall happiness and success. You can have a more balanced and satisfying existence if you set goals in more than one area.

2.4 Establishing Both Intermediate and Long-Term Objectives Achievable goals are the result of breaking them down into both long-term and short-term targets. One should have both long-term and short-term objectives; the former should paint a picture of your ideal future state, while the latter should lay out specific, attainable measures to get you there. Both are important if you want to keep moving forward and achieve your goals.

2.5 Conquering Difficulties and Problems There will be

difficulties and setbacks along the way as you pursue your dreams. But if you have the correct attitude and plan, you can conquer any obstacle. Master the art of overcoming obstacles by learning to see failures as stepping stones to success and by strengthening your resolve, resourcefulness, and perseverance.

2.6 Honoring Significant Achievers and Advancements

Take a moment to rejoice in the small victories along the road as you move closer to your big ambitions. Rejoice in the feeling of success that comes from getting closer to your goals, and give thanks for all your hard work and determination. You may keep yourself motivated and encouraged to keep climbing the ladder of success by rejoicing in your accomplishments.

2.7 Do Something: Make a Strategy for Your Goals Spend some time developing a strategy for achieving your unique set of

objectives before moving on. To make your aspirations a reality, you must first determine what is most important to you, then establish SMART goals, and last, create a plan of action. You will be prepared to begin the path to a meaningful and satisfying life with a well-defined strategy. ---
In this chapter, readers will learn how to make their dreams a reality by setting meaningful goals that are in line with their desires and using the tactics and tools provided.

- **CHAPTER 3: Crafting Your Daily Routine for Success**

Creating a Productive Daily Routine (Chapter 3) You can't build your life upon anything other than your everyday routine. Intentional daily rituals and habits are the building blocks of success, productivity, and general well-being, and we'll look at their significance in this chapter.

 3.1 Realizing the Influence of Habits The consistency, predictability, and forward motion that our daily routines offer is invaluable. They aid in time management, task prioritization, and maintaining concentration on what is important. You can maximize your productivity and build a life you love by making a routine that fits in with your values

3.2 Creating the Perfect Morning Schedule Start by seeing your perfect day unfold before your eyes. What would your ideal day consist of in terms of routines, habits, and activities? Make your routine work for you by including things like meditation and exercise first thing in the morning, setting up specific times during The day to work focused, and ending the day with relaxation and self-care.

3.3 Setting Priorities for Crucial Tasks You need to figure out what really matters if you want to be happy and successful in life. Some examples of such things are things having to do with health and fitness, self-improvement, professional and financial matters, interpersonal dynamics, and recreation. You may make sure that you're focusing on what's really important to you by making these things a daily priority in your routine.

3.4 Building a Modular Structure There should be some leeway in your daily schedule, but structure is still key. Any given day may bring its own set of challenges and unforeseen responsibilities. You can be calm and collected in the face of life's inevitable ups and downs if you make flexibility a regular part of your routine.

3.5 Integrating Reflection and Mindfulness

To develop presence, thankfulness, and self-awareness, incorporate periods of contemplation and mindfulness into your everyday life. If you're looking for a way to calm your racing thoughts and stay in the here and now despite the chaos of daily life, try writing, meditation, or even just taking a few deep breaths.

3.6 Making the Most of Your Time and Energy

Make a plan to be focused and productive all day long. Methods like time blocking, prioritizing tasks, reducing interruptions, and taking frequent breaks to regroup and concentrate are all part of this category. Make the most of every day and achieve your goals with more ease and joy by maximizing your concentration and efficiency.

3.7 Do Something: Create a Plan for Your Everyday Routine

Create a plan for your own daily routine before you go on. Create a framework that allows for development and adaptation by outlining the habits, rituals, and activities that will promote your success and well-being. You will be able to face each day with energy, purpose, and clarity when you use your daily routine as a map. --- Readers are given the power to create a daily routine that is in line with their values and goals in this chapter. It gives them the framework and the skills to achieve success, be productive, and feel fulfilled in their life.

ANALYZE YOUR THOUGHTS

- **CHAPTER 4: Creating Healthy Habits for Longevity**

Taking care of ourselves, both physically and mentally, is the first step towards living a happy and fulfilled life. Here we'll delve into the life-altering effects of developing routines that support health, vitality, and longevity.

4.1 The Value of Maintaining a Healthy Inhabits A robust and satisfying existence is built upon healthy behaviors. They improve our cerebral acuity, emotional fortitude, and general well-being in addition to our physical health. We may establish the groundwork for long-term health and longevity by making self-care a priority and embracing healthy lifestyle habits.

4.2 A Familiarity with the Science of Lifespan Investigate the science of longevity to learn what makes a person live a longer, healthier life. Gain insight into the most recent findings and evidence-based practices for enhancing health and vitality across the lifespan, including dietary habits, physical activity, stress reduction, and social interact want

4.3 Evaluate Your Present Practices Take stock of your present routines and decisions and think about how they affect your health. Take stock of your routines and determine which ones help you stay healthy and happy, and which ones could be holding you back from living the life you want.

4.4 Committing to a Lifestyle of Healthy Habits If you want to improve your health and happiness, you need to make a plan. If you want to live a long, healthy life, you need to make changes. These changes can be as simple as eating better, exercising more, getting more sleep, or learning to handle stress better.

4.5 Establishing Conscious Eating Practices Learn how to eat mindfully and reap the benefits to your health and life. Get in

touch with your body's signals
for when you're full and hungry,
eat slowly so you can fully enjoy
each bite, and learn to value the
healing potential of complete,
nutrient-dense meals.

4.6 Exercise and Physical
Activity Must Be Priorities Learn
how exercise and other forms of
regular physical activity can
improve your health and extend
your life. To improve your
energy, mood, and general
health, try out a variety of
movement styles that suit your

interests and preferences, and make exercise a daily part of your schedule. Supporting Psychological and Emotional Well-being

4.7 Take a look at ways to take care of your mental and emotional health, such meditation and mindfulness, doing things that make you happy and fulfilled, and making time for self-care and stress management a priority. If you want to succeed no matter what comes your way, you need to train yourself to be resilient, optimistic, and mentally strong.

4.8 Fostering an Encouragement-Filled Setting Take care of your health and happiness by surrounding yourself with positive people and things. Make an effort to surround yourself with supportive people who share your values of health and wellness, and do all you can to encourage good lifestyle choices and behaviors in your daily life.

- **CHAPTER 5: Cultivating Mindfulness and Mental Well-being**

Learning to Be Mindful and Taking Care of Your Mental Health Stress, anxiety, and other modern-day distractions may quickly take over a person's life if they let them. Our mental health can be greatly improved by the life-altering technique of mindfulness, which will be discussed in this chapter.

5.1 Getting a Hinge Around Mindfulness Being open, curious, and nonjudgmental while completely engrossed in the here and now is the essence of mindfulness. Meditation is not dwelling on the past or worrying about the future, but rather tuning into one's thoughts, feelings, and bodily sensations with openness and acceptance.

5.2 Advantages of Being Mindful Mindfulness has several positive effects on mental health, according to research. These include less stress, anxiety, and depression, better concentration and focus, better emotional control, and more resilience and happiness in general.

5.3 Making Mindfulness a Part of Everyday Living Find out how to bring mindfulness into your

everyday life in ways that are
both easy and effective.
Opportunities to cultivate
present-moment awareness can
be found throughout the day,
whether it's through formal
meditation techniques like
mindfulness meditation or body
scan exercises or casual practices
like mindful eating or walking.

5.4 Developing Self-Compassion
and Compassion for Others
Along with mindfulness, work on
becoming more empathetic and
compassionate. Be kind to

yourself and others around you by treating yourself with the same compassion, understanding, and love that you would give to a close friend. Increased resiliency, self-acceptance, and mental health can result from practicing self-compassion.

5.5 Overcoming Anxiety and Stress Master the art of mindfulness-based stress and anxiety management. To alleviate stress, unwind the body and mind, and find inner quiet, try mindfulness-based stress reduction (MBSR), progressive muscle relaxation (PRMS), or deep breathing exercises.

5.6 Developing an Attitude of Thanks and Appreciation

Gratitude and appreciation are powerful tools for developing mindfulness and enhancing happiness. Make it a habit to count your blessings—big and little—every day and to be grateful for all the good things in your life.

5.7 Taking Action: Making Mindfulness a Part of Your Daily

Life Do something specific to incorporate mindfulness into your everyday life before moving on. Begin by setting aside a small portion of your day for structured meditation, and as you become more accustomed to it, you can extend your mindfulness practice to incorporate more casual periods of being fully present in the here and now. Mindfulness and mental wellness are within your reach with regular practice and dedication. --- This brief chapter introduces readers to

mindfulness and offers practical
ways for enhancing mental well-
being, cultivating more
resilience, tranquilly, and
happiness via regular
mindfulness practice.

- **CHAPTER 6: Designing Your Dream Home Environment**

Beyond its practical functions, your home serves as an expression of your personality and a haven for your spirit. In this chapter, we will delve into the art of making your home a place that supports your health, encourages your imagination, and makes you feel at peace.

6.1 Establishing Your Goals

Start by picturing the perfect setting for your home. How would you like the mood to be set? Which styles, colors, and textures speak to you the most?

Give some thought to the type of house you see for yourself, whether it's a minimalist sanctuary, a chic urban hideaway, or a warm and welcoming hamlet.

6.2 Developing Ease of Use and Practicality Designing your home environment with comfort and usefulness in mind is essential. Think about how you want the room to look and how you want to live in it when you choose the furniture, decor, and arrangement. Make sure there are

quiet spots to unwind, ergonomic
desks for getting things done, and
common spaces for mingling.

6.3 Infusing of Individuality and
Significance Put your own spin
on things by decorating your
home with things that mean
something to you. Incorporate
pieces of your cultural
background, travel experiences,
and life journey into the fabric of
your home setting by displaying
treasured artwork, furnishings,
and relics that have personal

significance to you. Building Areas for Rest and Rejuvenation

6.4 Allocate specific areas of your home for unwinding and rejuvenation. Design a peaceful bedroom hideaway for a good night's sleep, a comfortable reading nook for some quiet time alone with your thoughts, or a peaceful meditation area for some quiet time alone with yourself. Bring in some greenery or other natural features to make people feel more at one with nature and help them relax.

6.5 Encouraging Welfare and Health Make your home a haven for health and wellness by optimizing its conditions. When designing a healthy and lively home, it's important to think about things like indoor vegetation, natural light, and air quality. If you want to improve your mental and physical health, you should install wellness amenities like a yoga studio, home gym, or a bathroom that feels like a spa. 6.6 Embracing Environmental Responsibility

and Long-Term Viability Think
about how your home design
decisions will affect the
environment and try to be as
sustainable and eco-friendly as
you can be. Reduce your carbon
footprint and make your home
more eco-conscious by installing
energy-efficient appliances,
using eco-friendly materials, and
practicing sustainable
construction.

6.7 Getting Started: Creating
Your Ideal House Create a
blueprint for your ideal house

before you go forward. Make use of home design periodicals and the internet as sources of inspiration, as well as to draught floor plans and vision boards. You may make your house a reflection of who you are by starting small and working your way up, room by room. --- In this brief chapter, readers will find ideas and advice for creating a house that is a reflection of who they are, what they value, and how they want to live their lives, all while fostering health, happiness, and environmental responsibility.

- **CHAPTER 7: Navigating Relationships for Happiness**

Having meaningful relationships with other people is essential to living a full life because they shape our happiness and the experiences we have. This chapter delves into the skill of cultivating deeper connections and better pleasure through navigating relationships with grace, empathy, and authenticity.

7.1 Developing an Awareness of Oneself Get a handle on your own wants, values, and relationship limits by working on your self-awareness. Take stock of your life so far, pattern it out, and figure out where you might improve. Having a solid grasp of who you are allows you to approach relationships with more authenticity, self-assurance, authenticity

7.2 Efficiently Expressing Yourself Relationships rely on communication because it lays the groundwork for intimacy, trust, and comprehension. For better connection building and conflict resolution, practice active listening, empathy, and honest communication. Open up about how you're feeling, what you need, and what you think in a kind and respectful way.

7.3 Establishing Appropriate Limits Protect yourself, your needs, and your principles by establishing healthy limits in your relationships. Make your boundaries known to others and be firm when you need to. In order to cultivate relationships that are healthy and respectful of each other, it is crucial to remember that setting boundaries is a kind of self-care and respect.

7.4 Developing a Heart for Others** Reach out to others and try to put yourself in their shoes;

this will help you develop compassion and empathy in your interactions. Put yourself in another person's position and try to understand things from their perspective to develop your empathy. Help those around you out by being kind, encouraging, and supportive, and do your best to provide a welcoming environment where people may feel comfortable being themselves and developing their potential. 7.5% Cultivating Positive Connections Spend effort cultivating positive, encouraging relationships that bring you up and motivate you. Put yourself in the company of like-minded individuals who will uphold your limits, encourage you to pursue your dreams, and share your beliefs. Build a broad group of supportive people around you—friends, family, and mentors—who can help you thrive.

7.6 Ending Negative Relationships When a relationship isn't helping you achieve your goals, it's time to break up. No matter the relationship you're in, whether it's a friendship, a love relationship, or a family dynamic, you should put your mental and emotional wellness first. With love and compassion, let go of poisonous relationships and have faith that better, more satisfying connections will replace the void.

7.7 Steps to Take: Nurturing Positive Relationships

Establishing and maintaining

positive relationships should be your top priority before moving further. Take stock of your present connections and think about how you may make them better. Be an engaged listener, establish reasonable limits, and put the people who make you happy, loved, and fulfilled first in your relationships. --- In order to help readers navigate relationships with more awareness, authenticity, and compassion—and therefore to foster deeper connections and

more happiness in their lives—
this brief chapter offers practical
advice and tactics.

- **CHAPTER 8: Balancing Work and Personal Life**

Finding a Healthy Work-Life Balance The key to happiness and success in life is finding a balance between your professional and personal responsibilities. To build a life that flourishes professionally and personally, we'll look at ways to strike a balance, establish boundaries, and put self-care first in this chapter.

8.1 The Work-Life Balance Concept Striking a balance

between your professional
responsibilities and the things
you enjoy doing and the people
you spend time with is what it
means to have a work-life
balance. Spending the same
amount of time on each activity
isn't the point; what's important
is figuring out what's most
important to you and focusing on
that. Eighth, Establishing Limits
You can save yourself time,
effort, and stress by drawing a
firm line between your
professional and personal lives.

Maintain a regular work schedule, avoid multitasking by not checking email or taking calls while on the clock, and establish clear boundaries with your superiors and coworkers to foster an environment of mutual respect and understanding.

8.3 Putting Yourself First You must make self-care a priority and an integral part of your daily schedule. Allocate time in your calendar to do things that make you happy and fulfilled, such resting, relaxing, and spending time with loved ones or engaging in hobbies and interests. In order to keep one's mental, emotional, and physical health in good shape, self-care is vital.

8.4 Making the Most of Your Time To make the most of your time and make room for other hobbies, optimize your productivity during work hours. In order to remain focused and effective, it is recommended to prioritize work, set attainable goals, and minimize distractions. To better organize your day and get more done, think about using time management strategies like the Pomodoro Technique or time blocking. 8.5 Developing Adaptability Keep an open mind about how you divide your time between work and play; you never know when one will demand more of your focus than the other. Maintain a flexible and resilient mindset; be ready to rearrange your priorities and timetable as circumstances demand.

8.6 Cultivating Relationships of Support Make an effort to surround yourself with encouraging people who will support your work-life balance goals. This can include friends, family, and coworkers. Find mentors or role models who have a good work-life balance and surround yourself with positive, encouraging people.

8.7 Taking Stock and Making Adjustments Take stock of your work-life balance on a regular basis, and if necessary, make changes to bring it in line with your priorities and principles. To build a life that is satisfying, long-lasting, and in sync with your career and personal aspirations, you must first take stock of what is going right and what could use some tweaking, and then be open to making some adjustments.

8.8 Developing a Strategy for a Healthy Work-Life Balance

Make a specific goal to achieve a healthy work-life balance before

moving forward. Maximize your
productivity and flexibility in
your business and personal life
by setting limits, prioritizing self-
care, and developing solutions. If
you put in the time and energy,
you can find a way to balance
your life so that you may succeed
in every aspect. --- In this brief
chapter, we provide readers some
practical advice and tactics for
balancing their personal and
professional lives so that they
can thrive in all areas.

- **CHAPTER 9: Financial Planning for a Secure Future**

Thoughts on Future Financial Security in Chapter 9 Being financially stable allows you to follow your heart and do what makes you happy, which is essential to living a full life. A solid financial foundation is essential to a comfortable retirement, and we'll go over some concrete steps to take in this chapter.

9.1 Acknowledging Financial Objectives First things first: figure out what you want out of life in terms of money. For you, what does a stable income mean? If you want to know how to save for retirement, purchase a house, have a family, or tour the world, you need to know what your short-term and long-term financial goals are

9.2 Planning for and Monitoring Spending To better understand your spending patterns and revenue streams, it is a good idea to make a budget. Determine how much money you need to spend on necessities, how much to put away, and how much to spend on pleasure, and see where you can make cuts or reallocate money so that you can reach your financial goals.

9.3 Establishing a Rainy-Day Fund Create a rainy-day fund to deal with unforeseen costs or financial difficulties. Put up enough money to cover three to six months of living expenses in a separate savings account. This will give you a cushion in case you lose your job, have a medical emergency, or anything else unexpected happens.

9.4 Prudently Handling Debt Make a plan to control your debt and pay as little interest as possible. Pay off high-interest debts first, such personal loans and credit card balances, and make a strategy to do so quickly. You can save money on interest and make payments easier by consolidating or refinancing coinsurance

9.5 Future-Proof Investments

To create money and ensure your financial stability in the future, you should investigate investment opportunities. Think about building a diverse portfolio that fits your risk appetite, investing horizon, and long-term objectives. Professional advice can help you make the most of your money in any investment vehicle—stocks, bonds, mutual funds, real estate, or retirement accounts—by reducing your exposure to risk and increasing your potential return.

9.6 Making a Retirement Plan If you want to retire comfortably and with peace of mind, you need to start saving now. Whenever feasible, put money into a 401(k) or individual retirement account (IRA) that your employer sponsors, and make sure to cash in on employer matching contributions. To create a retirement savings plan that fits your needs and fits in with your plans for the future, you might want to consult a financial counsellor.

9.7 Safeguarding Your Property
Get the right insurance to protect your family and possessions. To safeguard against unforeseen circumstances and reduce

financial risk, think about getting health, life, disability, and property and casualty insurance.

9.8 Ongoing Evaluation and Modification If your life or your financial objectives change, you should reevaluate your financial plan and make any necessary revisions. Be proactive in optimizing your financial strategy for long-term success and security by staying updated on economic trends, tax rules, and investment opportunities.

9.9 Practical Steps: Making a Budget

Get your individual financial strategy in order before you go ahead. Make a list of everything you need to accomplish, make a budget, put money aside for emergencies, and figure out how you'll handle debt, investments, retirement, and insurance. You may create a stable financial future that allows you to enjoy life according to your own standards with diligent planning and focused action. --- This chapter equips readers with the knowledge and tools they need to take charge of their financial destiny by outlining concrete steps for managing money, saving, investing, and preparing for insurance and retirement.

- **CONCLUSION: Sustainable Living**

Strategies for a Greener Tomorrow

Finally, "Sustainable Living Strategies for a Greener Tomorrow" provides a glimmer of optimism for the future of humankind's ability to live in peace with Mother Earth. We have set out on a life-altering journey through this book, seeking out creative solutions, inventive ideas, and ageless wisdom to help us live more sustainably. With this last page turned, may we take the lessons

learned and run with them,
resolving to be more
environmentally responsible,
more conscientious consumers,
and more aware of the significant
impact our actions have on the
planet in the future. No matter
how tiny, every action has the
potential to spark good change,
and with every eco-conscious
decision we make, we add to the
rich fabric of a greener future.
Join me on my journey towards a
better, more sustainable future,
where the natural world and

human ambitions coexist
harmoniously.

ANALYZE YOUR THOUGHTS

....

....

....

....

....

....

....

....

....

....

....

....

....

....

....